Apple Cider Vinegar Cures

Miracle Healers From The Kitchen

By

Sharon Daniels

Legal Disclaimers and Notices

Copyright © 2013 Sharon Daniels & Internet Niche Publishers- All rights reserved.

This book contains material protected under International and Federal Copyright laws and treaties. Any unauthorized reprint or use of this material is prohibited. Violators will be prosecuted to the fullest extent of the law.

The author, publishers and distributors of this product assume no responsibility for the use or misuse of this product, or for any physical or mental injury, damage and/or financial loss sustained to persons or property as a result of using this system.

The content of this book is for informational purpose only and use thereof is solely at your own risk. Readers should always consult with a physician before taking any actions of any kind relating to their health. The author, nor the publisher will in no way be held responsible for any reader who fails to do so. Any action taken based on these contents is at the sole discretion and liability of the reader.

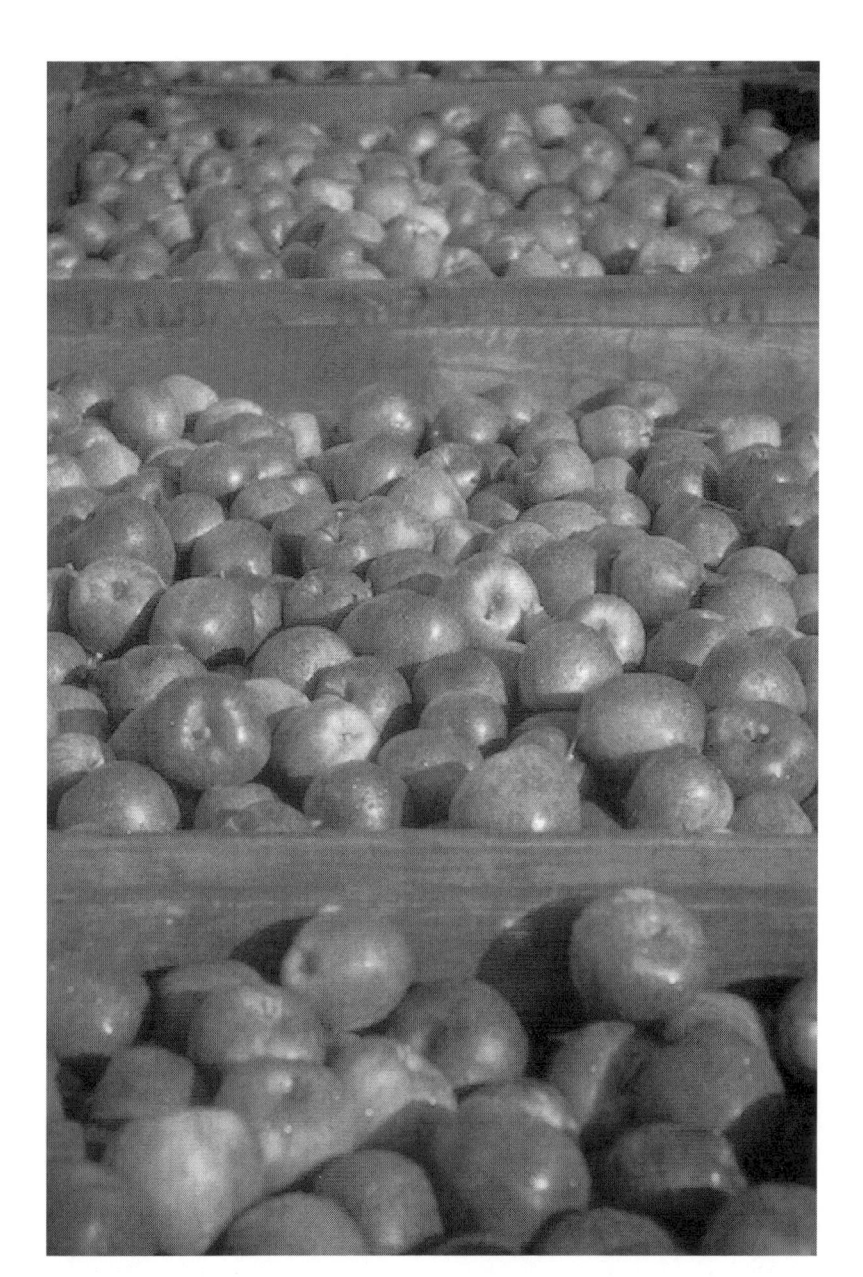

Contents

What is Apple Cider Vinegar? 8
    Cider vs. Juice 8
    What is vinegar? 9
    How does apple cider vinegar differ from other vinegars, and why does it matter? 10
    A Quick and Simple Apple Cider Vinegar Recipe 12
What Benefits Does Apple Cider Vinegar Provide? 13
What is Behind the Miracle? 14
Weight Loss 19
Diabetes 20
Atherosclerosis 21
Blood Pressure 21
Cholesterol 22
Osteoporosis, Arthritis and Other Bone-Related Conditions 22
Cancer 25
Bacterial Infections 27
    Ear Infections 27
    Food Poisoning Prevention 27
    Preventing and Treating Infections in Catheterized Patients 27
Fungal Infections 28
Sunburn 29
Hair Care 29
Nosebleeds 30
Stomach Upset 30
Pre-menstrual Syndrome (PMS) 31
Detox 32

Jellyfish Stings	33
Burns	34
Acne	34
Denture Cleaning	35
Precautions	35
Apple Cider Vinegar and Baking Soda	37
Apple Cider Vinegar and Water	38
Apple Cider Vinegar and Raw, Organic Honey	38
How it Works	39
Make Smart Meal Choices	41
Drink Your Way to Health	42
Dose as Needed	42
Pickle to Perfection	42
Poultry	43
Horses	44
Cattle	44
Sheep and Goats	44
Dogs and Cats	44
Making Herbal Tinctures	46
Insect Repellent	46
Household Uses for Apple Cider Vinegar	47
All purpose cleaning spray	47
Flea repellent	47
Ant deterrent	47
Fabric softener	48
Odor remover	48

Lime scale remover 48

Floor cleaner – even for delicate hardwoods 48

Drain cleaner 48

Cut flower food 49

Weed killer 49

Driveway spray 49

Gnat and fruit fly trap 49

Remove foul smells from your refrigerator 49

Clean your garbage disposal 49

Disinfect cutting boards 49

Polish brass, copper, pewter or steel 50

Clean gold jewelry 50

Remove odors and colors from hands while cooking 50

Disinfect produce 50

Unclog an iron 50

Enhance rinse cycles 50

Polish furniture 50

Remove pet stains and odor from carpets 51

Remove adhesives 51

References 52

Books 52

Medical and Scientific Journals 52

University and State Publications 53

Lay Science, Fitness, and Health Publications 54

Trade Publications and Patents 55

Introduction

Apple cider vinegar can do for you things that you would never expect from such an ordinary kitchen condiment. It's a safe, healthy, and nontoxic alternative to some of the most powerful disease-fighting drugs on the market.

In this book, I'll explain in detail exactly what apple cider vinegar can do for your health and wellbeing. I'll tell you why you should use apple cider vinegar, and explain how it's different from other types of vinegar. I'll make sure you handle the substance like a pro, so you don't have to worry about overdosing.

Best of all, I'll teach you how the apple cider vinegar can be a miracle for the health. You'll learn how to use apple cider vinegar to help fight extra weight, diabetes, high blood pressure and cholesterol, bacterial infections, sunburn, and much, much more!

I speak from personal experience when I tell you that apple cider vinegar changed my life. With the help of this book, and through the magic of this kitchen miracle, I hope your life will be changed in the same way.

Now, let's get started, shall we?

To your health,

Sharon Daniels

Why Apple Cider Vinegar?

There are many types of vinegar, made from nearly anything that can be fermented. Rice vinegar is especially popular in Asia, balsamic vinegar is a favorite in Italy, and white vinegar has been a kitchen staple in the United States for generations. What makes apple cider vinegar different enough to warrant its own book? In this chapter, we will discuss the health benefits and applications of apple cider vinegar, and what makes it a unique, powerful medicinal aid.

What is Apple Cider Vinegar?

Apple cider vinegar is vinegar made from apple cider. Simple enough, right? It might seem like it, but let's take a deeper look. What is apple cider? How does juice differ from cider? What is vinegar? How does vinegar made from apple cider differ from any other vinegar, and why does it matter? These are the questions we will address in this section.

Cider vs. Juice

Apple cider is made by mashing freshly washed whole apples, seeds and skin included, into a pulp that has the consistency of applesauce. This mixture is then carefully strained. The remaining liquid is apple cider – it's that easy! Unlike apple juice, apple cider is a raw product – true cider is not pasteurized. Apple juice is made by filtering cider to remove all solids, and is pasteurized. The shelf life of apple juice is often extended by vacuum sealing, adding sweeteners, and more filtering.

While the difference might seem minimal at first, the effect on the final product is distinct. Cider contains many nutritive properties that apple juice fails to provide. Pectin, found in apple skins, is present in apple cider. This substance has been shown to help keep serum cholesterol levels low. Apple cider is also a good source of potassium and iron, has no added sugars, and only 87 calories per glass. It must be refrigerated, or it begins to ferment.

Fermentation of apple juice takes significantly longer than the same process in apple cider. Apple juice becomes apple wine, and eventually apple vinegar – a rare product. Apple cider becomes hard apple cider – a popular alcoholic beverage in many English-speaking countries. Many countries in Latin America and Europe also have their own regional variations. The beverage takes 3 months-3 years to ferment, depending on temperature, components, and the specific recipe followed. In some parts of Europe and the United States, liquors may be made from double-distilled or triple-distilled hard cider.

Fermented apple cider eventually becomes apple cider vinegar. It is important to note that apple cider can be fermented to produce apple cider vinegar without much excess processing, and does not necessarily pass through a palatable hard apple cider stage before becoming vinegar. If you want to get the best nutritional value from your apple cider vinegar, you'll want an organic, unfiltered, apple cider vinegar that contains a substance called "the mother." We'll discuss this in greater detail in the next subsection.

What is vinegar?

The name vinegar literally means "sour wine." All vinegars are the product of a sugar-containing liquid that has been fermented with yeast and *acetobacter* bacteria. Before becoming vinegar, this sugar-containing liquid is an alcohol. This step is necessary, as the yeast and bacteria mixture work by converting the alcohol into the final vinegar product by producing acetic acid.

In the previous section, we mentioned "the mother"- this term refers to the film-like disc that forms on the top of fermenting vinegars. The mother is the yeast and bacteria colony. You may also hear this disc referred to as SCOBY or a "symbiotic colony of bacteria and yeast." If you have an older bottle of vinegar at home, "the mother" will naturally begin to form on the vinegar once it has been opened.

"The mother" is responsible for many of the health benefits associated with vinegar. The bacteria it contains help to eradicate harmful bacteria, especially in the digestive tract. This effect has been noted in chickens and other fowl as well as in humans. As a result, many chicken farmers actually add apple cider vinegar to their chickens' water!

The primary components of vinegar are acetic acid and water. The level of acid in most store-bought vinegars is 5-6%. Diluted acetic acid is not the same as vinegar, in part due to the absence of SCOBY. Federal law allows a substance to be labeled vinegar is if passes through the natural fermentation process which includes "the mother," and ranges in acidity from 4-7%. The nutritional properties of vinegar vary based on the starting material. Although SCOBY converts sugar to alcohol, and later to vinegar, it does not change the nutritional properties of the initial components. Vinegar made with nutritious ingredients that impart health benefits will provide those benefits, as well as those of "the mother" and of vinegar itself.

How does apple cider vinegar differ from other vinegars, and why does it matter?

Many of the health benefits of apple cider vinegar can be provided by other types of vinegar as well. This surprises many individuals, who assume that apple cider vinegar's status as a health food comes from numerous properties unique to this variety of vinegar. The truth is, however, that vinegar in general is very healthy! One of the primary reasons that apple cider vinegar is commonly used as a health supplement has to do with taste. This vinegar is very mild compared to many other common vinegars. Additionally, it has a pleasant aroma and taste when diluted into a tonic. It goes well with many types of fish and poultry, and can easily be made into salad dressings or even flavored vinegars.

There are some benefits to apple cider vinegar that are not found in many other vinegars. Earlier in the book we discussed the pectin and mineral content of apple cider, and its low calorie content. These are present in apple cider vinegar as well. Apple cider vinegar is lower in calories than many other vinegars, offers a lower glycemic load than balsamic vinegar – which is also known for its health properties – and is a very good source of manganese. In addition, apple cider vinegar may be more filling than other types of vinegar. Apple cider vinegar provides 2% of daily recommended calcium. The number might seem small, but vinegar also helps the body to absorb calcium, making its presence significant in this vinegar!

Apple cider vinegar is made by fermenting the juice of pulverized apples. Some processed versions of the condiment are created using evaporated apples or other apple derivatives. The processing differences can affect the nutritional and medicinal value of the final product, as can the quality of apples. This is important for several reasons. Since the skin of the apple is where many of the important components of apple cider vinegar originate, you want to have vinegar produced from an apple with a clean skin. While industrially produced apple ciders are made from washed apples, they still have pesticide residue. For this reason, organic apple cider vinegar is strongly recommended. The last thing you want in a daily health supplement is an unhealthy dose of pesticides.

Another important factor to consider when selecting an apple cider vinegar is pasteurization. When vinegars are pasteurized, it is not to prolong shelf life or food safety. The acidity of vinegar itself will take care of that. The goal is to kill "the mother," which gives the vinegar a clear, appealing appearance. For health purposes, you want "the mother," and a pasteurized apple cider vinegar works contrary to your goals!

If you can't find a good quality, organic, unpasteurized apple cider vinegar in your area, you can make one. There are several recipes available online for raw apple cider vinegar. All are fairly simple – essentially requiring nothing more than apples, apple cider, or a pre-made apple cider vinegar with juice, water, and "the mother." The process takes between 2 weeks and several months to complete, depending on the temperature and your SCOBY's growth rate. NEVER use homemade apple cider vinegar for pickling, however! This can be dangerous, as you have no way of knowing the acidity of your vinegar, which is a crucial factor in effective and safe pickling.

A Quick and Simple Apple Cider Vinegar Recipe

If you have an apple tree, it would be waste to buy apple cider vinegar. Homemade apple cider vinegar can be made with your favorite variety of apple, changing the final flavor to a product you find more appealing. There are many reasons why a homemade apple cider vinegar may be the best option for you. Making an apple cider vinegar from scratch – from apples or from cider – doesn't have to be a difficult process. There are some basic things to consider first, however.

1) Fall and winter apple varieties must be used to make apple cider vinegar! Other varieties don't contain enough sugar to produce usable vinegar. This means that green and yellow varieties and apples with a tart flavor should also be avoided in vinegar-making.
2) Metal containers will corrode during vinegar making. Use wood, glass, ceramic, plastic, enamel, or other non-metal containers to hold your vinegar while it ferments. Make sure that your containers are food-grade and sterile!
3) Do not use baking yeast to help the process along – **it doesn't work**. There are special species of yeast that are used to encourage fermentation. They can be obtained from wine-making supply stores or biological labs, but are not necessary. There is enough yeast in the air to begin the fermentation process. The addition of this specialized yeast will speed up the process, however.
4) When making vinegar, keep your fermenting solution between 60 and 80 degrees Fahrenheit.
5) As a general guide, if you want to yield 1 gallon of apple cider vinegar, you will need to use 20-25 lbs. of apples.
6) Cheesecloth is always good to have on hand for straining. If you don't have any, use a fine sieve.

Before you can make vinegar, you need to make cider. Wash all of your apples thoroughly, and remove the stems as well as any brown spots or bruises. Don't peel or core your apples, but do quarter them. If you have a juicer, you can run your apples through the machine to save yourself some time. Otherwise, you will need to manually crush and press your apples to yield the cider. Strain the mixture using the cheesecloth or sieve, letting the juice drain into your sterilized container(s).

If you are starting from cider, not the apples themselves, this is where you begin the process. If you have a wine-making yeast starter to use in your vinegar, add it now. Fill your container(s) ¾ of the way, and cover with cheesecloth or another breathable fabric. You want the yeast and bacteria to have access to oxygen, but you don't want flies in your vinegar!

Stir your soon-to-be vinegar in a dark location for 3-4 weeks, or until it begins to smell like vinegar. Don't be surprised or afraid if a little mold forms on top. The mother of vinegar will also be visible. Skim the mold off, but leave the mother (it will have a cellulose appearance and jelly-like texture). Taste-test your vinegar after it begins to smell until you have reached a flavor that appeals to you as a vinegar. As long as the mother of vinegar remains in the liquid and your vinegar is exposed to the air, fermentation will continue. It is important to note that homemade apple cider vinegar may vary widely in acid content, and may not be an effective cleaning agent. Homemade vinegar should not be used in canning, or in the preparation of foods that will be stored at room temperature.

What Benefits Does Apple Cider Vinegar Provide?

Apple cider vinegar has been a health remedy, recognized across cultures, for millennia. Medical studies and scientific investigations in recent years have disproven some widely held beliefs about apple cider vinegar's ability to cure nearly everything, while simultaneously proving the existence of some health benefits that were entirely unexpected. As you will see in the following chapter, apple cider vinegar is a powerful treatment for type 2 diabetes, lowers cholesterol, fights cancer, curbs appetite, helps prevent sudden blood sugar spikes, may increase dietary calcium absorption, kills many forms of harmful bacteria, and may prevent the build-up of fat stores in the body! There are many other health benefits that result from the use of apple cider vinegar. We will explore all of apple cider vinegar's **proven health benefits** in the next chapter.

In addition to its many health benefits, apple cider vinegar can be used to cure meats, and clean produce. We will delve into some of the many home uses of vinegars in the last chapter of this book.

What is Behind the Miracle?

There is no miracle. There *is* science! Vinegar's primary component, acetic acid, is a known component in the metabolism of carbohydrates and fats in the body. It is naturally present in the mucosal lubricant excreted in human and primate vaginas, where it serves an antibacterial – and interestingly enough, spermicidal - function. Acetic acid is also used to treat jellyfish stings, outer ear infections, and as a fungicide and antibacterial agent in numerous settings. The properties of acetic acid in more concentrated form become dangerous, and like all acids, it has to be handled with care. Vinegar, a dilute acetic acid, is generally considered harmless to humans, livestock and pets, but can still effectively accomplish many of the functions of more concentrated acetic acid solutions.

As we discussed earlier, the use of apple cider to make vinegar provides numerous health benefits. Pectin, a substance found in apple cider and the resulting vinegar, may help to lower cholesterol levels. The compound also helps to combat both diarrhea and constipation by altering stool consistency, and is a natural source of dietary fiber. The substance is commonly found in natural detox remedies, and after Chernobyl, was given to children from the area to help eliminate the radioactive cesium from their bodies!

In addition to pectin and acetic acid, apple cider vinegar also provides key minerals such as potassium and manganese. Potassium helps to facilitate nerve communication and response in the body, works to eliminate waste from cells, and combats the negative effects of sodium on blood pressure. Manganese performs important antioxidant functions in the body, and may help to manage conditions such as osteoporosis, arthritis, diabetes, PMS, and epilepsy. The mineral may also positively affect metabolism, bone development, and wound healing. Vinegar also contains numerous vitamins, polyphenolic compounds (polyphenols), mineral salts, and non-volatile organic acids!

Much of the available nutritional information on apple cider vinegar can be confusing – it's largely based on industrialized, pasteurized, distilled apple cider vinegar. Unfortunately, all that processing causes significant nutrient loss. Remember that RAW, ORGANIC, UNPROCESSED apple cider vinegar with "the mother" contains vitamins, minerals, and other beneficial compounds that are not found in processed varieties!

Apple cider vinegar isn't a miracle cure. It isn't a mysterious substance whose function is poorly understood overall. Although the action of its components in tandem is still being studied, it is composed of numerous substances that are known to provide health benefits. It's not really a surprise that apple cider vinegar has a positive effect on health and wellness when taken appropriately.

Myths about Apple Cider Vinegar

Apple cider vinegar has been the subject of much debate in recent years. Strong advocates of the condiment's nutritional applications argue that it is without dangers, while skeptics claim that it is without medicinal merit! Sadly, neither side is correct. The purpose of this book is to provide you, the reader, with sufficient and balanced information to decide if apple cider vinegar is right for you. We believe that its benefits outweigh its risks, and hope that you will feel the same way. Regardless of our stance on the substance however, real decisions can only be made with evidence. In this section, we will dispel some of the myths that circulate about apple cider vinegar – both bad and good.

Myth: Apple cider vinegar is a panacea, capable of treating nearly everything, without any negative effects.

Fact: Apple cider vinegar does offer significant health benefits, as we will discuss in the following chapter. There are drawbacks, however. It can't cure everything, and long-term use has been associated with significant and detrimental health consequences. Overuse of apple cider vinegar in the short term can also have significant negative ramifications. We'll discuss these in the next chapter in greater detail.

Myth: Apple cider vinegar is a common kitchen condiment, so it won't have any bad interactions with medication.

Fact: Apple cider vinegar, like many common kitchen ingredients, can interact negatively with some medications. Specifically, people taking Digoxin, Lanoxin, Thalitone, Diuril, HydroDiuril, Lasix, HCTZ, Microzide, insulin, water pills or diuretics should consult with a physician before consuming any quantity of apple cider vinegar, as negative reactions are possible.

Myth: Apple cider vinegar can't help with diabetes/Apple cider vinegar contains apple cider, so it is sweet and may cause blood sugar spikes.

Fact: Despite quite a few people trying to claim otherwise, apple cider vinegar can indeed help to control type 2 diabetes. There have been several studies in recent years, mostly coming from Japanese universities and institutions; that confirm apple cider vinegar's role in controlling or even reversing the condition. If you are currently being treated for type 2 diabetes, ask your doctor about the potential benefits of using apple cider vinegar. Your current medication doses might need to be adjusted if you wish to incorporate apple cider vinegar into your treatment plan, as it can potentially interfere with insulin, and is known to both lower blood sugar and prevent sudden blood sugar spikes! There is no sugar in apple cider vinegar – the natural sugars were converted to alcohol, which was later converted to acetic acid by "the mother."

Scientific Evidence for Healing With Apple Cider Vinegar

By now, you are surely curious about apple cider vinegar's healing abilities. In this section, we will discuss not only the medicinal properties of this common kitchen staple, but the studies and user testimonies that support these claims. After all, the facts are important! Additionally, we will go over some basic information about the potential side effects of apple cider vinegar when it is abused. The studies mentioned in this chapter are cited in the further reading section at the end of this book, so that you can do some more research yourself, and see how wonderful apple cider vinegar really is!

All of the information in this book is for your benefit as a consumer. The information presented is not designed to take the place of a doctor's advice, nor is it to be construed as medical advice. We just feel that it is important for everyone to know about the research regarding apple cider vinegar, and the good it can do for one's health Apple cider vinegar is an exciting substance that can truly help one live a healthier life! We are not, however, doctors or medical professionals.

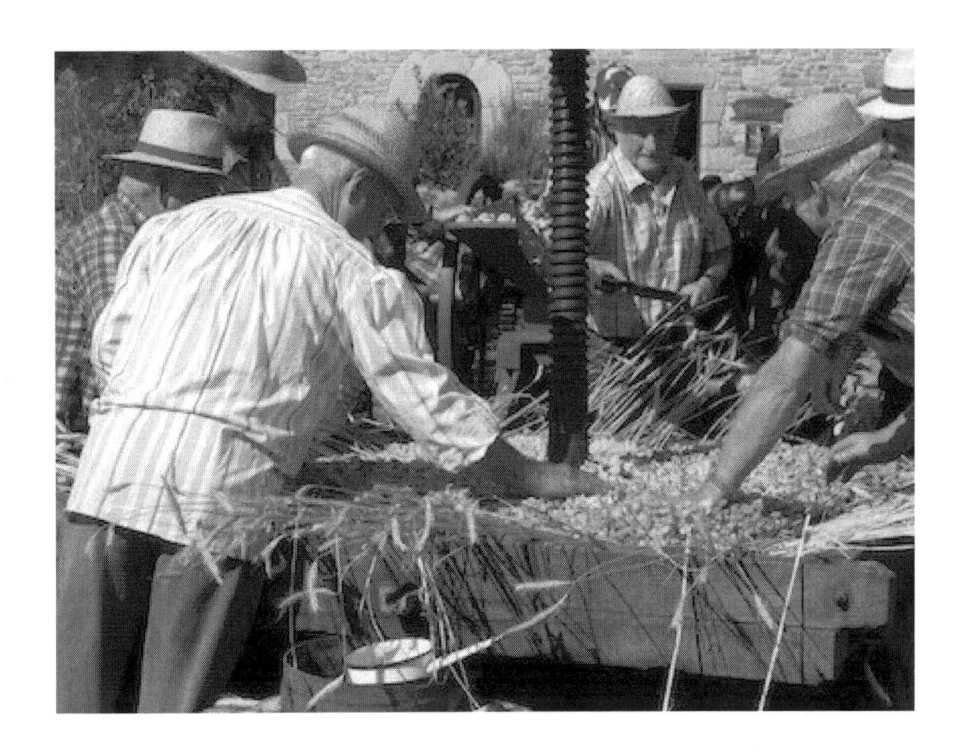

Weight Loss

Apple cider vinegar is a traditional weight loss remedy among some North African peoples. It has generally been used by women, and until recently the reasons for its effectiveness were unknown. There are actually several reasons why apple cider vinegar is effective at helping individuals lose weight, although its long-term use for this purpose is not recommended. Rather, apple cider vinegar is excellent at helping one lose weight initially, and to control appetite and keep weight off in the short term.

Apple cider vinegar can increase the feeling of fullness after a meal in healthy adult subjects. A 2005 study on women's caloric consumption indicated that a decrease of 11-16% in caloric consumption was noticeable on days when vinegar was included in the morning meal!

Vinegar is thought to slow the emptying of stomach contents, adding to a long-lasting feeling of satiety. There are mixed results on this effect in studies, however. Research is still ongoing regarding vinegar's ability to impact satiety.

A study on fat absorption in mice yielded results that could improve your waist line. Japanese researchers from the Central Research Institute of the Mizkan Group Corporation discovered that vinegar caused effects at the genetic level which led to 10% less fat gain in a group of mice who were fed vinegar vs. a control group. For a mouse, that might not be much – but think about what 10% of the average adult's body fat weighs – we're talking pounds, not ounces! Acetic acid and vinegar were theorized by the authors of this study to increase fatty oxidation and thermogenesis in the liver.

Diabetes

Vinegar was first studied in 1988 as a diabetes-fighting agent, although it's application as an antiglycemic agent dates to folk medicine from the 1800s, and perhaps even earlier! Since the late 1980's, numerous studies have confirmed that the substance is capable of assisting in diabetes management. There is some question as to how exactly vinegar is able to affect blood sugar absorption, gastric emptying rates, and glycemic response. What is known is that blood glycemic response slows significantly when vinegar is consumed, although this effect is nullified when baking soda is present. Interestingly, a 2001 study in the *American Journal of Clinical Nutrition* reported that the consumption of a single pickled cucumber with a meal may increase satiety and reduce the glycemic index of a meal by as much as 30%.

The antiglycemic function of vinegar has led some researchers and doctors to suggest that it may function similarly to Metformin or Acarbose, and sensitize the body to insulin over time. As a result, it is believed that vinegar consumption might be able to slow the progression to diabetes in individuals who are at a high-risk for developing the condition. Vinegar's behavior as a diabetes fighting agent is still going on, although results to date are promising. In a few years, doctors might even be prescribing set doses of apple cider vinegar, in lieu of diabetes management medications!

Atherosclerosis

Atherosclerosis is a condition in which the inside of the arteries of a mammal develop fatty plaque deposits. The condition is often related to high cholesterol, and may lead to significant risk for heart disease and stroke. A study conducted in 2011 showed that vinegar has the ability to reduce the number of atherosclerotic lesions in the aorta of rabbits with high cholesterol. In short, this means that the number of dangerous fatty deposits in the largest artery connected to the heart had fewer deposits of fatty plaque, and the risk of heart disease was therefore lowered in rabbits that consumed vinegar as a part of their diet. While testing in human subjects has not been performed to date, this research shows strong possibilities for applications in human atherosclerosis treatment as well.

The authors of the study noted that diets high in fruits and vegetables with high levels of polyphenolic compounds have been tied to a reduced risk for atherosclerosis. Vinegar is high in polyphenols, and varieties such as apple cider vinegar, with especially potent levels of these compounds, may be especially useful in combating atherosclerosis! In addition to removing existing plaque buildup, vinegar may reduce the likelihood of atherosclerosis by lowering cholesterol levels. This will be discussed in greater detail below.

Blood Pressure

Studies conducted by Japanese researchers in 2001, 2003, and 2009 revealed that vinegar lowers blood pressure in hypertensive individuals. The methodology and sample seizes of these studies do lead to questions regarding the validity of results, however. Despite the potential problems with study design, similar results have been observed by numerous researchers working with laboratory animals. In all cases, it appears that the active agent for lowering blood pressure is the acetic acid present in vinegar. In vinegars with higher polyphenol content, these compounds may also play a beneficial role. Apple cider vinegar provides the benefits of both – think of it as two dietary supplements in one! The hypotensive effects of vinegar may be amplified if dried bonito is consumed with the vinegar.

Cholesterol

A 2008 Scientific American blog post reported on an experiment conducted by two sisters on high cholesterol treatment with apple cider vinegar, a remedy their Middle Eastern grandmother had advocated for years. The results of their study demonstrated that the pectin in apple cider vinegar is beneficial in lowering cholesterol levels, to at least a small degree. Numerous studies conducted on laboratory rats and mice have yielded mixed results regarding the effects of apple cider vinegar on lipid profiles, however.

Tests using diluted acetic acid on rats demonstrate that acetic acid is capable of preventing hyperlipidaemia (high cholesterol). Based on the above information, there is reason to suspect that the combined effects of pectin and acetic acid in apple cider vinegar may help to lower overall cholesterol serum profiles. Investigations into the effects of apple cider vinegar on cholesterol levels are ongoing.

Osteoporosis, Arthritis and Other Bone-Related Conditions

The jury is still out where the treatment of bone conditions with apple cider vinegar is concerned. Depending on the quality, production method, and nutritional content of the apple cider vinegar being used, it can contain bone-building minerals such as potassium and calcium. Highly processed vinegars and those with longer fermentation periods are much less likely to retain these components, however. Studies that have been conducted using apple cider vinegar have yielded mixed results. If you want to help save your bones, use only RAW, ORGANIC, UNPROCESSED apple cider vinegar!

Individuals who consume apple cider vinegar in high quantities for a long period of time are actually susceptible to *bone loss*. As scary as that might sound, there are reasons to think that apple cider vinegar can be beneficial in treating bone loss, osteoporosis, arthritis and other bone-related conditions. For example, acetic acid, the primary component of apple cider vinegar, and all vinegars for that matter, is an acid. Acids in general help the body absorb nutrients more readily, including those used to maintain bone health and density. Think of apple cider vinegar as your mineral supplement's best friend. By consuming vinegar with your bone medicines, you can ensure that your body absorbs more of the vital nutrients and minerals it needs to build strong bones and prevent further bone loss!

A 1984 study of rats with adjuvant arthritis revealed no arthritis or inflammation reducing effects from apple cider vinegar consumption. More recently, however, an evaluation of chronic pain and inflammation symptoms resulting from arthritis was conducted on laboratory mice and rats in Iran. This 2004 study revealed that mice and rats suffering from sciatic nerve ligation improved significantly, in a dose-dependent manner, when given apple cider vinegar! The researchers proposed that the B vitamins found in apple cider vinegar may be at least partially responsible for the pain-relieving and anti-inflammatory effects observed in the study. They recommended further study of the interaction of apple cider vinegar on arthritic inflammation and pain, although to date no further studies have been conducted.

In 2008, Sir Ranulph Fiennes, a renowned explorer and adventurer who has run 7 marathons in 7 countries in 7 days, among other feats, reported his family's success with apple cider vinegar as a treatment for osteoarthritis. He reported that both he and his mother defeated arthritis pain by consuming honeygar - a honey and vinegar mixture - on a daily basis, following a strict diet regimen, bathing in Epsom salts, and taking mineral supplements. His belief is that the vinegar and honey mixture is responsible for his pain relief. A church organist in England reported similar results. Once bedridden for severe arthritis pain, and unable to play the organ, she has returned to an active and happy lifestyle with the help of apple cider vinegar and honey! Several similar anecdotal accounts are available on-line, and are largely tied to the work of a British nurse in 1961. The nurse conquered her own rheumatoid arthritis using the same honey and vinegar regimen, and opened an institute to help others using her cure.

The use of vinegar as a treatment for arthritic pain is common in folk medicine around the globe. Modern personal accounts, some scientific investigations, and historic evidence suggest that vinegar has a role in reducing arthritic pain. Apple cider vinegar seems to be particularly effective. The mechanism behind the remedy is not well understood, but will hopefully be uncovered through future medical inquiries.

Individuals suffering from other bone and rheumatic conditions may wish to take apple cider vinegar with care, and consult frequently with their general practitioner or osteopath, in order to make sure that bone loss is not resulting from overconsumption of the vinegar. Balance is important – remember, it is always possible to have too much of a good thing! While it appears to be an effective remedy that can help relieve pain and inflammation while helping bone growth when taken in moderation, larger doses may result in the opposite effect.

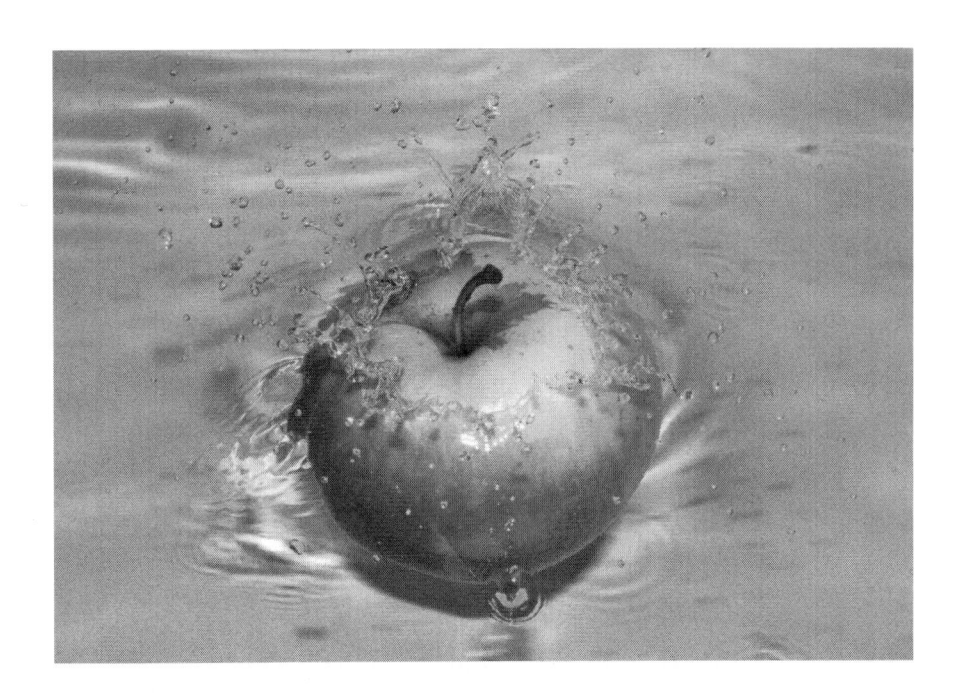

Cancer

Several studies in both lab rats and humans have revealed cancer-fighting properties of vinegar. The studies were done using rice vinegar and sugar cane vinegar, but the cancer-growth inhibiting function of vinegar is believed to be primarily the result of the acetic acid content of vinegar. This implies that apple cider vinegar may provide the same benefit. In tests, rats that were 'given' sarcoma or colon tumor cells and consumed a diet which contained vinegar showed decreased tumor size and growth when compared with a control group that did not consume vinegar. Additionally, the addition of vinegar to the diet also stimulated natural cancer-killing cells in the body!

The creation of short chain fatty acids as a result of the acetic acid's conversion to acetate in the stomach, and acetate's role in short chain fatty acid production, are thought to be at least partially responsible for the effectiveness of vinegar in fighting colon cancer in humans. Research is still being actively conducted in this area.

According to a 2004 study in the journal *Biofactors*, in vitro application of vinegar caused apoptosis in human leukemia cells. In China, a 2003 study on vinegar ingestion showed a decreased risk for esophageal cancer. Care should be taken by individuals with bladder cancer and other urinary tract cancers, however. A Serbian study published in 2004 showed an increased risk for bladder cancer among individuals who regularly consumed vinegar.

Another cancer fighting feature of vinegar is its polyphenol content – these compounds fight oxidative stress in plants, and work as antioxidants in humans as well. Their antioxidant role is crucial to battling cancer as well as fighting heart disease. While there are types of vinegar with higher polyphenol content than apple cider vinegar (kibizu and Kurosu), they are generally more difficult to come by and more expensive.

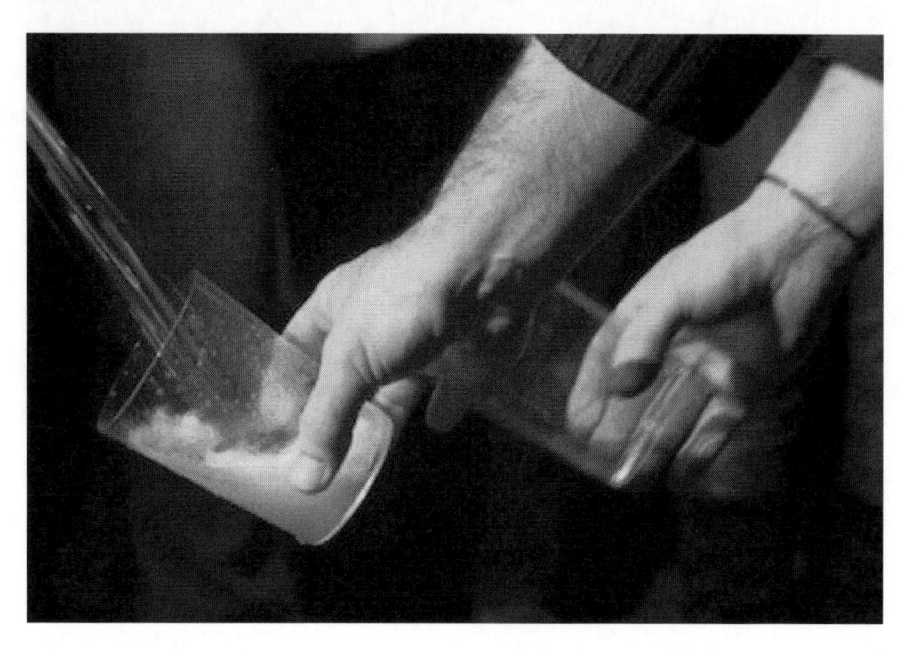

Bacterial Infections

Ear Infections

Individuals who frequently suffer from ear infections may be happy to hear of a cure they probably haven't tried – a diluted vinegar rinse! Apple cider vinegar's acetic acid concentration is normally 5-6%. To treat an ear infection with a warm water and vinegar rinse, a 2% acetic acid solution is recommended. Higher acid content can damage the ear, so if you choose to try this remedy, be sure to dilute the rinse carefully. The mixture is effective at treating otitis media, otitis externa, and granular myringitis, and several studies have reported its success in treating both children and adults.

Food Poisoning Prevention

A 2007 study published in the Journal of Food Protection reported that vinegar with a 5% acetic acid content – apple cider vinegar contains 5-6% acetic acid – is an effective bactericidal agent. The bacteria which were killed using 5% acetic acid vinegar were *S. aureus, L. monocytogenes, S. Enteritidis, E. Coli 0157:H7, S. sonnei* and *Yersinia* species. In layman's terms – the bacteria responsible for many food-borne illnesses and severe food poisoning! Cooking with vinegar and using vinegar-based salad dressings may help to prevent infections with these bacteria.

Preventing and Treating Infections in Catheterized Patients

A study on the effects of vinegar consumption and the resulting frequency of urinary tract infections in individuals who required long term catheterization revealed that vinegar fights, and may prevent, urinary tract infections! The study was conducted using rice vinegar, but may hold true for all types of vinegar, as acetic acid is believed to be the component in vinegar which kills bacteria. Further study is needed on this topic, but the results are promising. It is important to note that most urinary tract infections are caused by *E. coli*, bacteria which vinegar is known to kill.

A 2001 study, conducted in Hong Kong, demonstrated the ability of vinegar to combat difficult to kill bacterial infections that occurred following peritoneal dialysis. Researchers used distilled white vinegar with a pH of 3 in combination with Ciprofloxacin to treat infection with *Pseudomona aeruginosa*, a particularly difficult to kill and rapidly colonizing bacteria that often occurs at the site of peritoneal catheter exits. The treatment was 97% effective, with no return of the bacteria – significantly better than historical controls using standard treatment modalities! The pH of the vinegar is thought to be the primary agent responsible for the effectiveness of this treatment, suggesting that other vinegars, including apple cider vinegar, may be able to provide similar antibacterial effects.

Fungal Infections

Vinegar is known to have antifungal properties. In organic farming, it is sometimes applied to fruits or vegetables to prevent the formation of fungi, but can also kill plants in high concentrations, so its use is limited. In humans, it has long been touted as a folk remedy for yeast infections, nail fungus, and jock itch! The actual medical literature says surprisingly little about this remedy, however.

One available study of the effectiveness of apple cider vinegar on inhibiting fungal growth was conducted at Thi Qar University in 2011. The researchers discovered that for the treatment of outer ear fungal infections such as otomycosis, apple cider vinegar is an effective remedy. The vinegar inhibits the growth of numerous fungal species, including *Candida albicans, Aspergillus niger, Aspergillus flavus*, and *non-Candida albicans*. The concentration used in the study was 5% acetic acid, but no dosage was determined for topical application. Undiluted vinegar is highly acidic and can burn the skin and damage the ear canal. Caution is advised when using apple cider vinegar as a topical remedy for fungal infections, as a result. Concentrations high enough to kill fungi may also damage skin in sensitive individuals. The authors of the study recommend additional testing to determine appropriate dosing.

Minor fungal skin infections may be easily treated with apple cider vinegar in diluted form, as listed in this book for the treatment of bacterial ear infections, as well. If you have a minor topical fungal infection, try dabbing a little on a cotton ball, and apply directly to the affected site. If you have sensitive skin, dilute the vinegar with distilled water beforehand. According to The Doctors Book of Home Remedies, some physicians in the United States advocate the practice of applying apple cider vinegar to topical fungal infections much as one would apply alcohol topically – including for swimmer's ear.

Sunburn

Ever get a sunburn so bad that just moving was painful? Most people will try anything to get rid of the pain of bad sunburn, but extreme measures aren't necessary. The answer is in the pantry! A cool vinegar and water bath may help to ease sunburn discomfort. A full bath with 1 cup of vinegar added should be enough to do the trick. Make sure to apply lotion afterwards, however. Vinegar can be drying, which will aggravate the sunburn in the long run if you fail to moisturize. This remedy comes from a suggestion by Dr. Carl Korn, former dermatology faculty member at the University of Southern California.

Hair Care

In The Doctors Book of Home Remedies, apple cider vinegar is proposed as a remedy for excessively oily hair. Kirsten Hudson, a health and beauty expert for Huffington Post and OrganicAuthority.com, advocates its use for shine and texture. An apple cider vinegar and water rinse (1:1 ratio) creates shine naturally by closing the cuticle, which makes the hair reflect more light. Let the mixture sit for a few minutes, and rinse to remove the vinegar smell. Daily use is not recommended, due to the acidic nature of apple cider vinegar. Use it like a hot oil treatment – once a week will leave you with fabulously shiny, soft and gorgeous locks. The best part is that this remedy works for ALL hair types!

The antimicrobial properties of apple cider vinegar may also help to improve scalp health and combat dandruff. A 2011 study on herbal remedies for dandruff published in the International Research Journal of Pharmacy (India) found apple cider vinegar to be an effective method of treatment for this condition. It may take up to 8 weeks to function, and dandruff may recur later, however.

Nosebleeds

Otolaryngologyst Dr. Jerold J. Principato recommends inserting a cotton ball that has been dipped in vinegar into the nose to help stop excessive bleeding. The remedy works due to the acid content of vinegar – it helps to cauterize the wound that is bleeding, while also cleaning it. According to Health911.com, a leading natural health and wellness site, drinking a solution of apple cider vinegar in water may also be beneficial. This may be related to apple cider vinegar's ability to fight hypertension, as well as its antioxidant and polyphenol content. Antioxidants have been shown to help prevent nosebleeds, and nosebleeds are often a symptom of hypertension. The reason might not be clear, but the remedy works!

Stomach Upset

When mixed with raw honey, apple cider vinegar is a common folk remedy for heartburn, indigestion, and stomach discomfort related to over-indulgence. Dr. Deborah Gordon recommends the remedy on her website, http://www.drdeborahmd.com, and lists a preference for Manuka honey's use whenever possible. Who knew an acid could cure indigestion?!

Pre-menstrual Syndrome (PMS)

Many of the symptoms of pre-menstrual syndrome can be addressed with apple cider vinegar supplementation. Vinegar is a natural diuretic, and is used in detox treatments as a result of this property. One of the primary problems which cause PMS complaints is water retention. Women experience headaches, irritability, bloating and gastrointestinal upset as a result of excess fluid retention. As a result, many common over the counter treatments for PMS include caffeine as a diuretic. Apart from being addictive, many people just can't handle caffeine, or have been told by their doctor that they need to avoid it. Apple cider vinegar is a healthy alternative to a painkiller and caffeine cocktail!

A common complaint of women suffering from PMS is increased acne due to hormone fluctuations. As we will discuss later in this chapter, apple cider can be used as an astringent to relieve acne. Additionally, the mineral content of apple cider vinegar includes calcium and magnesium, as well as B vitamins! These vitamins and minerals are frequently given to women suffering from PMS to help alleviate their symptoms. In short, apple cider vinegar offers many benefits for women suffering from discomforts caused by PMS.

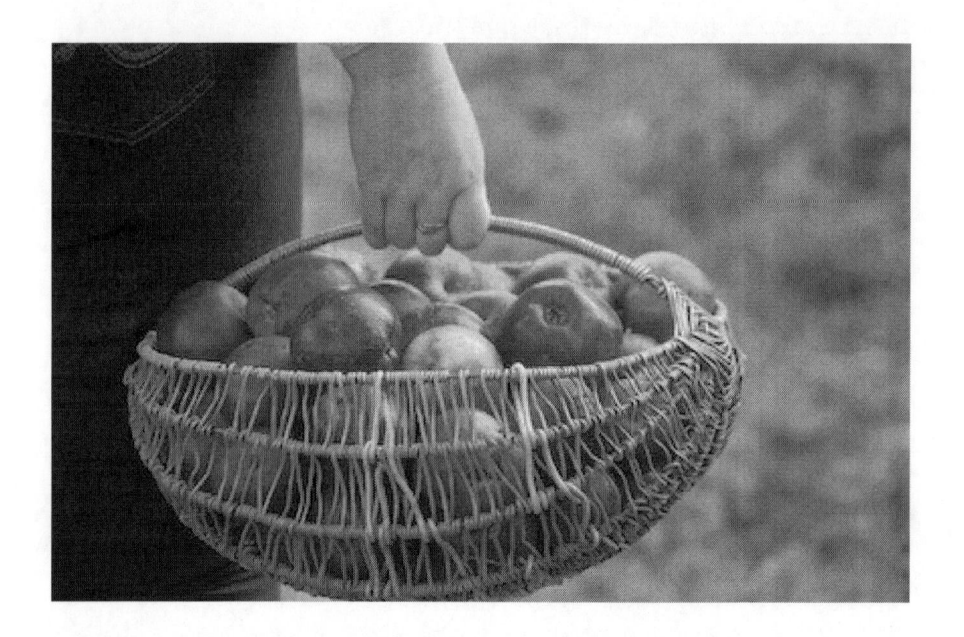

Detox

As a nutritional concept, detox is not recognized outside of alternative medicine communities. There are many aspects of detox which are inherently good for the human body, however, and apple cider vinegar is an excellent agent in achieving many of the desired effects. First and foremost, many of vinegars components are known to be involved in water balance in the body. As we discussed earlier in this book, they also play a key role in removing waste from cells. Healthier cells make a healthier body. After all, if the parts aren't, how can the whole organism be healthy?

Short term and alternate-day fasting has been associated with numerous health benefits. In three studies conducted in the past decade, cancer treatment outcomes improve with alternate day and short-term fasting. Chemotherapy treatments have also been more successful when combined with fasting. Caloric restriction is a reliable life-extending measure, even in healthy individuals, and fasting appears to offer the same benefits. Laboratory animals have been shown to live 40% longer as a result of caloric restriction alone! Insulin sensitivity and resistance to diabetes also improves as a result of fasting. So how does this relate to detox and apple cider vinegar?

Healthy fasting strategies are commonly used as part of detox programs. Some popular detox cleanses or diets include the use of apple cider vinegar. Apple cider vinegar is effective for more than one reason – in addition to containing components which remove cellular waste, vinegar also helps to keep the bowels moving at a safe and regular pace. The substance also decreases appetite, making the process of fasting easier. Dieters who have tried apple cider vinegar detox cleanses complain about the taste, but revel in the energy provided by apple cider vinegar - cleanses don't always include outright fasting, but caloric restriction is almost always present. A little apple cider vinegar diluted in water and taken after every meal is one common cleanse with reportedly good results. One of the reasons this cleanse is preferred is the vitamin and mineral content of apple cider vinegar. The condiment is a natural energy shot, due to the rich content of vitamins, minerals, organic acids and polyphenolic compounds it provides. It is crucial to note that pasteurized, filtered apple cider vinegar does not contain the trace minerals, vitamins, enzymes and beneficial bacteria found in raw, organic, unfiltered apple cider vinegar!

Jellyfish Stings

The most effective treatment for jellyfish stings of all types is hot water. This deactivates jellyfish venom, and makes it innocuous to humans. If you're at the beach, however, hot water can be hard to come by. One supply to always have on hand is a small bottle of apple cider vinegar. The acetic acid in the vinegar deactivates the nematocysts of jellyfish venom. This remedy is particularly effective when dealing with box jellyfish such as *Chironex fleckeri*. If you cannot immediately immerse the sting in hot water, coat it with apple cider vinegar and head to the nearest hospital for further evaluation. Some jellyfish stings can be deadly, or cause lifelong pain and paralysis if left untreated.

Burns

Dr. David J. Hufford of Penn State University advocates using a 1:1 vinegar and water mixture on minor burns, including those caused by concrete. Vinegar works by neutralizing the agent causing the burn, and hence is most effective in the treatment of minor alkaline chemical burns. In addition to its application in treating sunburns and minor chemical burns, the acetic acid in vinegar is especially effective at killing bacteria that are commonly found near the site of severe burns. The application of apple cider vinegar to severe burns should be carefully discussed with your physician, however.

In 2003 a study conducted on lab rats revealed that a 5% solution of acetic acid – roughly the same amount as found in apple cider vinegar – was not only effective at neutralizing the agent responsible for alkaline chemical burns, it also reduced the damage and improved healing time. Although commonly advised, rinsing the burns with water was not as effective as treatment with the acetic acid solution. Once again, vinegar's merit was noted by modern medical investigation!

Acne

According to a letter in the professional journal Our Dermatology Online, hyperpigmentation following severe acne can be remedied using vinegar to help increase the pace of natural exfoliation. Individuals suffering from active acne infections may also find vinegar to be a useful astringent. It is recommended for topical use in a 1:1 diluted solution with water that can be applied similarly to other acid astringents to decrease the severity of acne infection. If you are being treated for acne, consult with your dermatologist prior to use, in order to prevent interactions with other topical medications. Say goodbye to expensive medications and over the counter creams and cleansers – this cheap household remedy is all you need to banish your acne!

Denture Cleaning

Unlike commercial cleaners, dentures cleaned with vinegar do not damage the mucosal tissue, but are cleaned effectively. A study published in the Journal of Contemporary Dental Practice in the year 2000 suggested vinegar as a safe, reliable, denture-cleaning liquid.

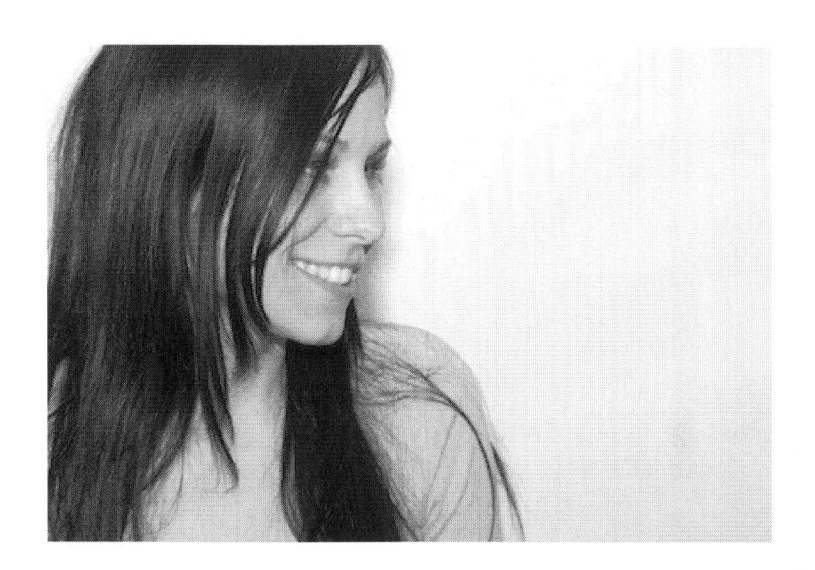

Precautions

As with most health supplements, there are some side effects to the use of apple cider vinegar. The information in this sub-section is based on scientific observation and patient files, and should be weighed carefully before you begin an apple cider vinegar regimen. Apple cider vinegar is a powerful acid, and as such can have some significant complications if mishandled or overused.

Apple cider vinegar tablets should be avoided. One of the beneficial substances in raw, organic, apple cider vinegar is "mother of vinegar," *acetobacter* bacteria which help convert sugars into alcohol, and alcohol into acetic acid. These are not present in distilled apple cider vinegar or in apple cider vinegar tablets. Additionally, since apple cider vinegar tablets ulated, the actual content of the pills may vary significantly brand. One study examined the contents of multiple brands t they differed significantly from each other and from the ingredient lists provided on their packages. In one particularly unpleasant incident, an Australian woman suffered esophageal burns and required medical care after an apple cider vinegar tablet became lodged in her throat. She continued to experience pain and difficulty swallowing for 6 months following the incident.

Long-term use of apple cider vinegar in high doses has been linked to hyperkalemia, hyperreninemia, and osteoporosis. Potassium levels in the body can be lowered by long-term consumption of vinegar, although raw, organic, apple cider vinegar may contain enough potassium to offset this effect. The same cannot be said for distilled apple cider vinegar, as both distillation and pasteurization break down vital nutrients and minerals. These are potentially serious complications, and shouldn't be taken lightly. Use apple cider vinegar in healthy moderation, and avoid distilled, non-organic versions.

Patients with kidney problems or diabetes should discuss their use of apple cider vinegar as a remedy with their treating physicians. Hypoglycemia and kidney complications are possible side effects of apple cider vinegar use, and the liquid can also interfere with some medications prescribed for these conditions.

Alkalizing Your Body with Apple Cider Vinegar

There are many individuals who believe in the medicinal value of alkalizing the body with a combination of apple cider vinegar and baking soda. This combination is thought to help relieve a wide variety of ailments, including anxiety, irritability, headache, sore throat, excess mucous production, nasal and sinus infections, and decreased energy.

Blood pH is normally between 7.35-7.45, slightly alkaline. Proponents of the alkaline-acid diet believe that one should aim to consume foods with a pH equal to that of human blood. Eating a diet high in acid leads to the development of numerous health problems, including the ones listed in the preceding sentences. Despite apple cider vinegar's status as an acidic food, it is thought to help restore the alkaline-acid balance in the body and is frequently prescribed by alternative medicine practitioners for this purpose.

Although this use for apple cider vinegar hasn't been thoroughly researched, many individuals on alkaline-acid balancing diets swear by the effectiveness of apple cider vinegar. It may be that, as with many other types of folk medicine, science has yet to catch up with popular knowledge, and in a few short years there will be numerous studies confirming the alkaline-acid balancing ability of vinegar.

We have included three popular alkalizing remedies in this section. Although designed and commonly used by homeopathic and naturopathic healers for alkaline-acid balancing effects, these tonics are also an excellent way to include apple cider vinegar in your daily diet.

Apple Cider Vinegar and Baking Soda

Many of the beneficial effects of apple cider vinegar on blood sugar are diminished or eliminated when it is combined with baking soda. As a result, if your health goals involve blood sugar maintenance, do not use this preparation. pH balancing effects remain the same, however, so don't worry if that is your goal.

Mix 2 tablespoons of apple cider vinegar with ¼ teaspoon of baking soda. Take this mixture 2-3 times per day on an empty stomach. Users claim that this preparation provides a little extra energy boost to help you get through the day, too. Be careful not to use this preparation in the long term, unless further diluted with water. Damage to tooth enamel and the soft tissues of the mouth is possible due to the high acid content of the vinegar, and the chemical reaction taking place between the baking soda and vinegar while the mixture is being consumed.

Apple Cider Vinegar and Water

Probably the most popular detox tonic, apple cider vinegar and water safely dilutes the vinegar without compromising its beneficial effects.

Mix 1 teaspoon - 2 tablespoons of raw, organic, apple cider vinegar with 8 ounces of water. Drink immediately. Drink this mixture daily to improve overall health.

Apple Cider Vinegar and Raw, Organic Honey

Apple cider vinegar and honey is a tasty treat with an extra benefit – if you use raw, organic honey that is produced in your local area, you are decreasing your likelihood of seasonal allergies each time you take the tonic. Honey contains small traces of local pollens. As a result, it functions similarly to allergy shots, by desensitizing immune response to pollens. If you are a highly allergic individual, or are currently experiencing allergy symptoms, do not begin taking this formulation.

Mix 2-4 tablespoons of apple cider vinegar with 1-2 tablespoons of honey. Dilute the mixture in 8 oz. of distilled water and drink after every meal. You can also make a gallon of this mixture ahead of time, using the same proportions, and refrigerate it for convenience. Remember to shake before consuming, however. Otherwise, the mother will settle to the bottom of the mixture.

How it Works

Apple cider vinegar is an effective alkalizing remedy for the body due to the way that our bodies use the substance. Although it enters the body as an acid, the digestion process converts apple cider vinegar into an alkaline substance, and it helps to regulate the body's pH as a result. Many individuals test their urinary pH in order to see how the vinegar works. This can be helpful, but it doesn't fully convince many skeptics. As the common saying goes, the proof is in the pudding. If you have any doubts about the effectiveness of apple cider vinegar, try it. There are thousands of accounts of success with this remedy on the internet, and you will find that resources such as www.earthclinic.com contain message boards where individuals share their success stories.

A friend of mine has a daughter who was very ill. Modern medicine was having difficulty addressing her condition, and essentially suggested that my friend and his wife give up on their precious little girl. Obviously, as concerned parents, they couldn't do that. They sought the help of a naturopath, who suggested that an alkaline diet might benefit their child. One of the top recommendations that they were given was to give their daughter apple cider vinegar every morning in the baking soda and vinegar preparation. Just a few short weeks later, their baby girl was back to normal – her painful suffering was alleviated, and my friend and his wife relaxed in the knowledge that she is ok. Today, the entire family uses apple cider vinegar to maintain an alkaline pH, and have also made some other dietary modifications, such as limiting their consumption of meat, in order to keep their bodies healthy.

My own case is not as grave as their little girl's, but I suffer from extreme allergies. Urinary pH during allergy attacks changes, and as a result, my allergist recommended that I try apple cider vinegar as a dietary supplement to help prevent attacks. I tried allergy shots beforehand, and they weren't working – my only other alternative was a steroid injection every 6 months. Since I have an extreme fear of needles, I complied with the apple cider vinegar suggestion. I find the honey preparation easier to handle than the other two forms, and so added it to my diet last year. The results have been amazing – despite high pollen counts in my area, and less time to clean (which means more dust mites), I have been able to breathe much easier this year. The benefits of this remedy were perfect for me, as I started taking it during the winter, when my allergies are mildest. The combined effects of honey and apple cider vinegar have kept me from turning to my inhaler for emergency relief, although I still carry it. I feel miles better, and have even been able to venture outdoors and enjoy the countryside, instead of hiding myself away in the house on high pollen count days.

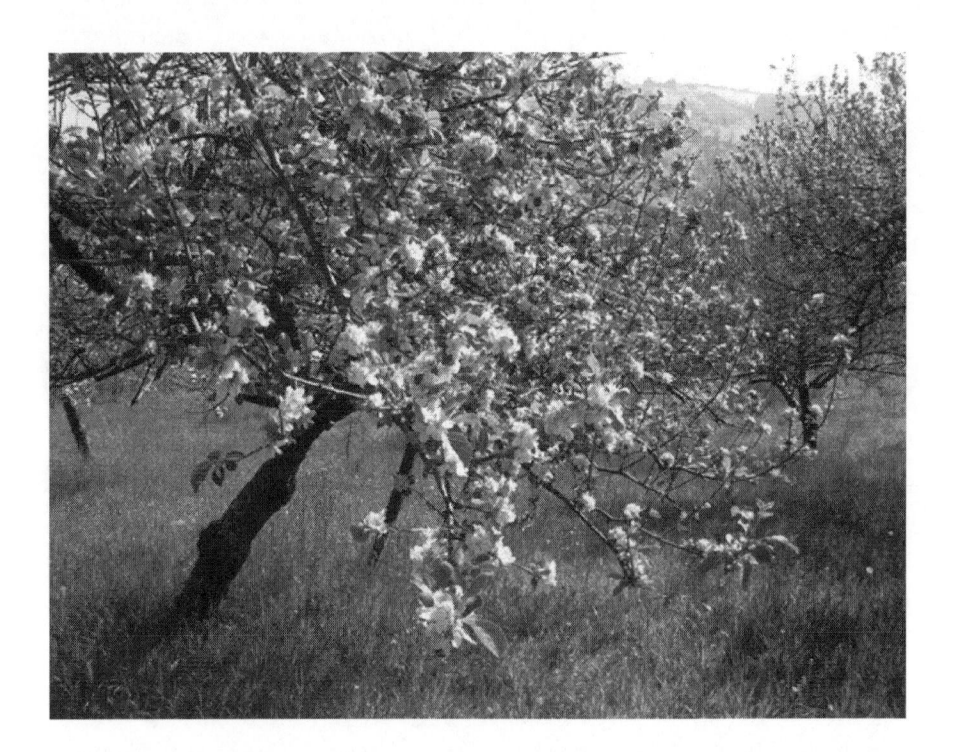

How to Add Apple Cider Vinegar into Your Life

Are you interested in adding apple cider vinegar to your life in a healthy and productive manner? The use of this substance as a common kitchen condiment makes it an easy addition to most diets! In this chapter, we will go over a few basic steps you can take to make apple cider vinegar a part of your daily care rituals, and your diet.

Make Smart Meal Choices

Vinegar is in many of our foods. It is a key component of mayonnaise, takes a lead role in most salad dressings, and is perfect for marinating chicken. Vinegar also can be reduced with sugar to produce sweet glazes for cooked vegetable dishes, and is added in the last few minutes of cooking to many soups, helping to round out flavor profiles. Many Asian cuisines incorporate vinegar on a regular basis, and sauces such as ketchup and mustard would be lost without it.

Read the ingredient labels of your family's favorite condiments. Homemade alternatives are better than processed foods in terms of flavor and health, for numerous reasons. Processed foods are generally higher in sodium and lower in nutritional value than their homemade counterparts. When you prepare your own mustard, ketchup, or barbecue sauce, you can customize the flavor to what your family prefers. Salad dressings are a breeze, and chances are that your family has a recipe for grandmom's favorite marinade or dressing floating around. Now is the time to use it! Make your own mayonnaise, salad dressings, sauces, soups, and other items that would normally contain vinegar using apple cider vinegar instead. You won't be sorry.

Drink Your Way to Health

One of the easiest ways to consume apple cider vinegar is to prepare a tonic with it. Use one of the recipes for alkalizing your body – preferably the one with honey and water, for honey's extra health benefits – and enjoy it half an hour before every meal.

Another way to drink apple cider vinegar is to mix 1-2 teaspoons with apple cider. The flavor is nice and juice-like, with just a little extra kick. Even the youngest members of your family will enjoy apple cider vinegar with cider. They probably won't even notice the difference between it and regular juice!

Dose as Needed

You can make apple cider vinegar a part of your daily diet, or you can consume it as needed. If you are suffering from a short-term condition that apple cider vinegar treats, use the information in the previous chapter, and take apple cider vinegar as needed to resolve your complaint.

Pickle to Perfection

If you are into home canning and pickling, substitute commercially-produced, raw, organic apple cider vinegar for ordinary distilled vinegar in your canning recipes. You can also make table pickles by lightly spritzing vegetables with spices and apple cider vinegar.

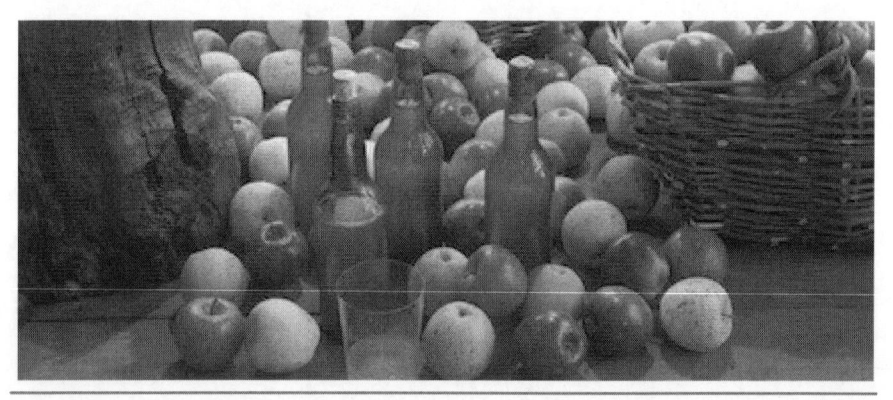

Apple Cider Vinegar for Your Pets and Livestock

The health and beauty benefits of apple cider vinegar aren't limited to human use. Apple cider vinegar is commonly employed on farms and by veterinarians to help domestic animals thrive. Poultry farmers, horse owners, and pet lovers everywhere should be aware of the benefits of this substance for their animals. In this chapter, we'll go over some of the most common uses of apple cider vinegar in animal care. Remember that vinegar is an acid, and should always be diluted for use with animals. Specific remedies for veterinary conditions are readily available on-line, but should be discussed on a case-by-case basis with your veterinarian before use. The tips below are not meant to substitute for a veterinary opinion – they are based from personal testimony, livestock, and veterinary medicine publications targeted towards a lay audience.

Poultry

According to Homestead Organics, apple cider vinegar offers numerous benefits for poultry – more than for any other type of livestock, in fact. The liquid can reduce the odor of feces, reduce bleeding from minor injuries, relieve itchy skin or feather problems, control pain and encourage wound healing, and control or eradicate internal parasites and infections. Additionally, when fed to egg layers, apple cider vinegar can increase fertility and stamina, while helping hens produce eggs with stronger shells. The use of apple cider vinegar in poultry may also improve feather health and overall immune system function. The substance works by lowering stress levels, improving appetite and digestion, and helping the body break down and process vital nutrients, fats, and minerals. When added to water feeders, it can also prevent the growth of algae and reduce the frequency of necessary cleaning. Do not use in metal feeders, as the acid will lead to corrosion.

Horses

Like dogs, horses can become a part of one's family over time. When a horse falls ill, it can be a saddening experience. Apple cider vinegar can help prevent painful intestinal stones in these gentle ruminators, and can also improve hoof health. For insect prone areas, owners will be happy to note that apple cider vinegar also works as an insect repellent for horses.

Cattle

Homestead Organics reports that the use of apple cider vinegar in dairy cattle diets can prevent difficult births and increase milk production. The condiment is also said to improve curdling in the maw and rennet-bag, and reduces the somatic cell count. Common infections such as mastitis, milk fever, anemia and ringworm can also be treated with apple cider vinegar.

Sheep and Goats

Farmers who keep sheep and goats for wool and pelts will be happy to learn that apple cider vinegar can improve wool quality. The occurrence of kidney stones and urinary calculi can be reduced by the use of apple cider vinegar as a supplement in these animals' feeds or water. Remember to not use metal feeders, as the acetic acid can cause metal to corrode.

Dogs and Cats

We mentioned that apple cider vinegar can be an effective insect repellent – including for fleas – earlier in this book. Let's take a closer look at how it can help your four legged friends. Hot spots on dogs can be treated by applying apple cider vinegar topically. Ringworm and itchy skin can be treated in a similar manner, although you might want to check with your vet first, to make sure that they are up to date on your pet's health problem.

Your dog and cat may produce urine that burns your lawn or stains the carpets in your home. Tear trails, little brown streaks extending from your dog's eyes, can be prevented, as can damage to lawns and carpets. Add a little apple cider vinegar to your pet's water bowl, and the problems should clear up on their own. The extra bonus, of course, is that you won't have to clean the water bowl as often – the apple cider vinegar will take care of that for you! Increasing your pet's water intake can also help with the aforementioned problems when combined with apple cider vinegar use.

If your pet is prone to kidney stones, ask your vet about supplementation with apple cider vinegar in their water bowl. A little apple cider added to their daily water may help to prevent stone formation – especially in cats. Adding a few drops to a dog's ears post-grooming may help clean them and prevent infections, but as with humans, make sure to dilute the vinegar! If your pet has a poor appetite, add a little bit of apple cider vinegar to their kibble or wet food. It can encourage appetite, and provide a change in flavor that they find appealing.

Dogs suffering from arthritis may fair well with apple cider vinegar supplementation. The condiment also appears to generally improve overall health and wellness in domestic animals. Apple cider vinegar supplementation may also reduce tooth decay and nail splitting in dogs.

Other Uses for Apple Cider Vinegar

Making Herbal Tinctures

There are many uses for apple cider vinegar outside of the realms of beauty, supplement, and animal care. One of these is the creation of herbal tinctures. Individuals who use herbal medicines often incorporate tinctures into their medicine cabinet. In most cases, tinctures are prepared with a strong alcohol such as vodka. For people who wish to avoid any and all alcohol – for religious, lifestyle, or other reasons – this can be problematic. By preparing tinctures with apple cider vinegar, however, the use of alcohol can be avoided.

In order to prepare an herbal tincture, you will need a large quantity of the herb you wish to make the tincture from, apple cider vinegar, and a dark, sterile, glass jar with a lid that can be tightly sealed. Put your herbs - preferably dried, but if not, thoroughly washed – into the glass jar until it is mostly full. Cover the herbs with apple cider vinegar. Seal jar. Every day for two weeks, shake the jar vigorously for several minutes. After two weeks, strain the mixture. The tincture is ready for use, and can be rebottled into small, tightly-sealed eyedropper jars and stored until needed. Tinctures have a nearly indefinite shelf life if stored properly, although they are most effective when used within 5 years.

Insect Repellent

Many individuals who are eco-conscious do not wish to use insect repellents. There are numerous natural remedy recipes available on-line, some of which are for insect repellents made from apple cider vinegar. You don't really have to go to much effort in making a bug repellent from apple cider vinegar, however. If you use 2 tablespoons of vinegar in your daily diet, the smell of your sweat won't be as appealing, and most species of fly and mosquitoes will leave you alone!

If you want a bug repellent spray, try making an herbal tincture with apple cider vinegar, parsley, sage, rosemary and thyme. Dilute your tincture with ½ water, and spray before heading out. You might not smell too good while the mixture is wet, but it is effective. There are certain species of fly that are attracted to the smell of apple cider vinegar, however, so the best method is actually ingesting the vinegar! The mixture works best for mosquitoes. Adding lemongrass to the tincture may increase its effectiveness.

Household Uses for Apple Cider Vinegar

Apple cider vinegar can do as much for your home as it can for your pet and you! Today's cleaning supplies often include toxic chemicals or allergens. Many individuals are also concerned about the negative effects of these chemical solutions on the planet, as well. In order to avid damage to yourself or the Earth, try the following household tips for apple cider vinegar use. You'll be surprised how much the substance can do, and by the fact that it has largely been relegated to the kitchen in recent years!

All purpose cleaning spray

½ cup apple cider vinegar mixed with 1 cup of water can be used to effectively clean and sanitize windows, glass, mirrors, bathroom tiles, and kitchen surfaces, including microwaves and ceramic oven tops.

Flea repellent

If you have pets, and your pets have fleas, it can seem impossible to get rid of the tiny pests. Spray your pets, furniture, carpets, and any surfaces where you have seen fleas with a 1:1 mixture of apple cider vinegar and water to chase them away from your home and animals.

Ant deterrent

If your house has an ant problem with change of seasons, confuse them by spraying apple cider vinegar over their food trails. The scout ants will lose their path, and not be able to return to the colony to report that they found food in your home. Occasionally the vinegar also kills the ants.

Fabric softener

Add ½ cup of apple cider vinegar to your washing machine with the detergent, and you'll emerge with soft clothing, less static, and no need for laundry sheets, which are believed to be carcinogenic, and contain allergens that irritate some individuals.

Odor remover

Ok, vinegar is smelly, as everyone knows. When it dries, however, the odor dissipates. Apple cider vinegar's acetic acid content helps it to kill odor causing bacteria, so use it as a substitute for air fresheners. When it dries, all you will smell is a nice, clean home.

Lime scale remover

Apple cider vinegar's acidic components eat through lime scale with ease, making it an excellent, non-toxic alternative to commercial lime scale removers!

Floor cleaner – even for delicate hardwoods

Mix 1 cup of apple cider vinegar into 1 gallon of warm water and use to clean floors. Remember to mop up excess water and vinegar mixture, so that the floor isn't damaged.

Drain cleaner

Mix ½ cup of baking soda and ½ cup of salt together. Pour this powder down the partially-clogged drain. Follow by pouring ½ cup of apple cider vinegar down the drain. The components react to produce carbon dioxide, a harmless gas. Industrial and commercially available versions can produce toxic gas fumes, and can also harm pipes. This mixture is gentle and non-toxic.

Cut flower food
Mix 1 teaspoon of apple cider vinegar with 1 teaspoon of raw sugar. Add to a vase of cut flowers to extend their lifespan.

Weed killer
Applied directly to common weeds in the garden, vinegar is an effective herbicide. Most weeds will die if their leaves are sprayed with the substance. For tough to kill plants, inject apple cider vinegar directly into the roots.

Driveway spray
Apply apple cider vinegar to driveways and sidewalks to return original color, prevent weed growth, and repel insects.

Gnat and fruit fly trap
Mix 4 cups water, 2 tbsp. sugar, 2 tbsp. apple cider vinegar, and 1 tsp. of dish soap together. Leave this mixture in your kitchen, or wherever you have the fruit fly problem, and the insects will naturally be drawn to it. Eliminate any other potential food sources in the area, to ensure success.

Remove foul smells from your refrigerator
Place a small glass filled with apple cider vinegar in your fridge. It will trap the odors within 48 hours.

Clean your garbage disposal
Make ice cubes with 1:1 apple cider vinegar and water mix. Toss into garbage disposal and crush as needed in order to clean the disposal and remove foul odors.

Disinfect cutting boards

Wipe your cutting boards with full strength apple cider vinegar. Spray the cutting boards with 3% hydrogen peroxide afterwards, and wipe dry.

Polish brass, copper, pewter or steel
Mix ½ cup apple cider vinegar with ½ teaspoon of salt. Add unbleached flour until you have a smooth paste. Apply to metals and let sit for 15 minutes. Wipe clean, rinse, and polish dry. Steel can be cleaned by applying vinegar solution directly to the surface and immediately polishing dry.

Clean gold jewelry
Submerge in apple cider vinegar for 10-15 minutes, remove, rinse and polish dry.

Remove odors and colors from hands while cooking
Rinse hands with apple cider vinegar to remove the smell of garlic or onion, or the dyes from beets and berries.

Disinfect produce
Wash fruits and vegetables with a mix of 8 parts water to 1 part vinegar in order to kill bacteria and clean your produce.

Unclog an iron
Add vinegar to a mostly full iron, and run on steam setting for 5-7 minutes. Unplug, cool, drain and rinse 2-3 times to remove vinegar smell.

Enhance rinse cycles
In both the laundry machine and dishwasher, adding ½-1 cup of apple cider vinegar to the wash process will decrease the amount of soap residue from washing, and leave clothes and dishes cleaner and brighter.

Polish furniture

Use a mixture of 1 part olive or linseed oil and 1 part apple cider vinegar to polish wood furniture. Test first, to ensure color-fastness of furniture finishes.

Remove pet stains and odor from carpets
Apply 1:1 water and vinegar to carpet working from the center of a pet stain to the outside with a sponge. Clean with this mixture until stain is gone. This method can also help to deter future pet potty accidents.

Remove adhesives
Apply apple cider vinegar directly to adhesive residue from price tags, or even bumper stickers in order to remove the residue.

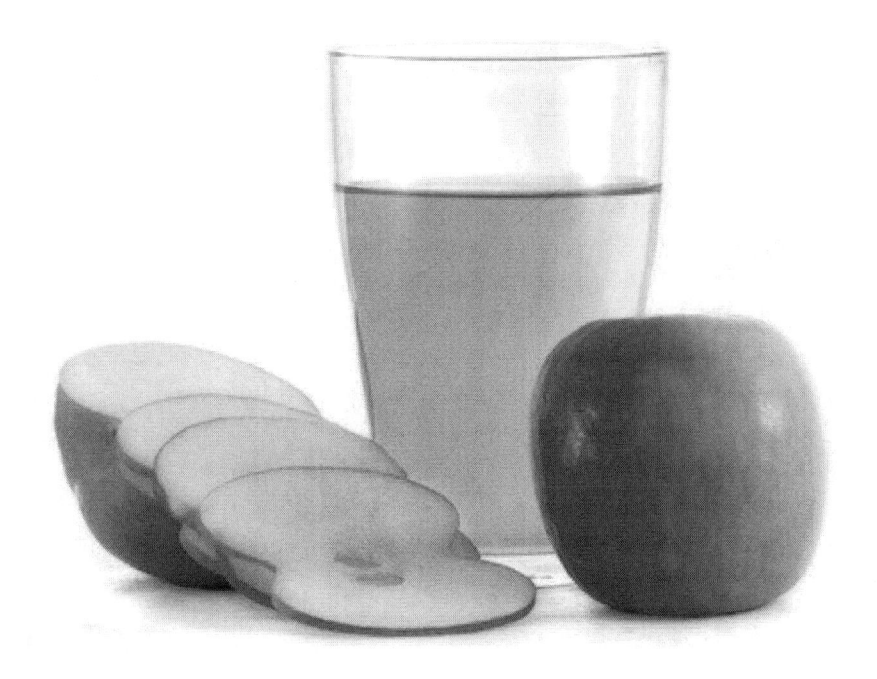

References

Books

1) The Doctor's Book of Home Remedies, Edited by Debora Tkac, Bantam Books, 1991, New York
2) Cooking Ingredients, Christine Ingram, Hermes House, 2008, London

Medical and Scientific Journals

1) http://www.ncbi.nlm.nih.gov/pmc/articles/PMC1785201/
2) http://www.journals.elsevierhealth.com/periodicals/yjada/article/S0002-8223(05)00477-3/abstract
3) http://www.andjrnl.org/article/S2212-2672(12)00943-4/abstract
4) http://www.ncbi.nlm.nih.gov/pubmed/23373303
5) http://journal.muq.ac.ir/en/index.php/jmuqen/article/view/214
6) http://brn.sagepub.com/content/14/3/294.short
7) http://www.ncbi.nlm.nih.gov/pubmed/22980269
8) http://www.ncbi.nlm.nih.gov/pubmed?term=apple%20cider%20vinegar&itool=QuerySuggestion
9) http://www.ncbi.nlm.nih.gov/pubmed/12167888
10) http://www.ncbi.nlm.nih.gov/pubmed/11893257
11) http://www.ncbi.nlm.nih.gov/pubmed/8694129
12) http://www.ncbi.nlm.nih.gov/pubmed/12690268
13) http://www.ncbi.nlm.nih.gov/pubmed/15630262/
14) http://www.ncbi.nlm.nih.gov/pubmed/15149153/
15) http://www.ncbi.nlm.nih.gov/pubmed/15489210/
16) http://www.ncbi.nlm.nih.gov/pubmed/15612246/
17) http://www.ncbi.nlm.nih.gov/pubmed/12468628/
18) http://www.ncbi.nlm.nih.gov/pubmed/12875624/
19) http://www.ncbi.nlm.nih.gov/pubmed/15237578/
20) http://www.ncbi.nlm.nih.gov/pubmed/16015276
21) http://www.ncbi.nlm.nih.gov/pubmed/16321601/

22) http://www.academicjournals.org/jmpr/pdf/pdf2011/4May/Setorki%20et%20al..pdf
23) http://www.ncbi.nlm.nih.gov/pubmed/9858130
24) http://www.ncbi.nlm.nih.gov/pubmed/14745664
25) http://www.ncbi.nlm.nih.gov/pubmed/11826965
26) http://www.ncbi.nlm.nih.gov/pmc/articles/PMC2704332/
27) http://pubchem.ncbi.nlm.nih.gov/summary/summary.cgi?cid=176#x94
28) http://www.journal.su.ac.th/index.php/suij/article/viewFile/48/48
29) http://www.nlm.nih.gov/medlineplus/potassium.html
30) http://journals.cambridge.org/download.php?file=%2FBJN%2FBJN95_05%2FS000711450600119Xa.pdf&code=3847dc8d6c9c6f9ee5fb4dfe7e2a40f0
31) http://ijpr.sbmu.ac.ir/?_action=articleInfo&article=466
32) http://www.ncbi.nlm.nih.gov/pubmed/12711953
33) http://www.odermatol.com/wp-content/uploads/2011/09/15.Post-Acne-Hyperpig.pdf
34) http://www.sciencedirect.com/science/article/pii/S1561541309600557
35) http://www.nature.com/onc/journal/v30/n30/full/onc201191a.html
36) http://www.irjponline.com/admin/php/uploads/vol-issue3/3.pdf
37) http://www.nlm.nih.gov/medlineplus/ency/article/001505.htm
38) http://www.sci.sjp.ac.lk/ojs/index.php/fesympo/article/view/192
39) http://stm.sciencemag.org/content/4/124/124ra27.full.html
40) http://impactaging.com/papers/v1/n12/full/100114.html
41) http://www.potravinarstvo.com/journal1/index.php/potravinarstvo/article/viewArticle/156
42) http://repository.thiqaruni.org/TMJ-2011-1/16.doc

University and State Publications

1) http://cardinalscholar.bsu.edu/handle/123456789/195877
2) http://www.ext.colostate.edu/pubs/foodnut/09355.html
3) http://www.umm.edu/altmed/articles/manganese-000314.htm

4) http://ohioline.osu.edu/hyg-fact/5000/pdf/5346.pdf
5) http://lpi.oregonstate.edu/infocenter/minerals/manganese/
6) http://www.mass.gov/agr/massgrown/cider_juice_difference.htm

Lay Science, Fitness, and Health Publications

1) http://www.webmd.com/diet/apple-cider-vinegar
2) http://www.naturalnews.com/035997_apple_cider_vinegar_remedies_health.html
3) http://www.lifesciencesite.com/lsj/life0904/360_10755life0904_2431_2440.pdf
4) http://altmedicine.about.com/od/applecidervinegardiet/a/applecidervineg.htm
5) http://healthybliss.net/benefits-of-raw-apple-cider-vinegar/
6) http://www.benefits-of-honey.com/vinegar-and-honey.html
7) http://www.naturalstandard.com/news/news200507032.asp
8) http://www.clarksnutrition.com/ns/DisplayMonograph.asp?DocID=bottomline-applecidervinegar&storeID=2691B1FE187D41ACB869A85CA5957A0A
9) http://nutritiondata.self.com/facts/spices-and-herbs/217/2
10) http://www.naturalnews.com/031969_apple_pectin_radiation.html
11) http://www.webmd.com/vitamins-supplements/ingredientmono-500-PECTIN.aspx?activeIngredientId=500&activeIngredientName=PECTIN
12) http://www.versatilevinegar.org/researchnews.html
13) http://www.scientificamerican.com/blog/post.cfm?id=need-to-lower-cholesterol-try-apple
14) http://www.care2.com/greenliving/apple-cider-vinegar-miracle-for-home-and-body.html
15) http://www.homesteadorganics.ca/vinegar_apple_cider.aspx
16) http://www.dirtdoctor.com/Vinegar-Apple-Cider-Vinegar-Cures_vq2365.htm

17) http://www.organic-pet-digest.com/benefits-of-apple-cider-vinegar.html
18) http://www.dailymail.co.uk/health/article-37317/The-healing-powers-vinegar.html
19) http://www.ask-curtis.com/can-applying-vinegar-neutralize-a-skin-burn-from-concrete/
20) http://www.dailymail.co.uk/health/article-1053045/Sir-Ranulph-Fiennes-I-beat-arthritis-vinegar-cure-passed-mother.html
21) http://www.telegraph.co.uk/news/newstopics/howaboutthat/6949863/Vinegar-cures-church-organist-of-crippling-arthritis-pain.html
22) http://www.huffingtonpost.com/organic-authoritycom/apple-cider-vinegar-beauty_b_1924171.html
23) http://www.naturalnews.com/038131_apple_cider_vinegar_hair_treatment.html
24) http://www.health911.com/nosebleeds
25) http://www.drdeborahmd.com/solutions-acute-indigestion
26) http://health.howstuffworks.com/wellness/natural-medicine/home-remedies/home-remedies-for-burns1.htm
27) http://www.refinery29.com/juice-cleanse-detox-weight-loss?page=2
28) http://www.grit.com/the-chicken-chick/make-raw-apple-cider-vinegar-acv-with-the-mother-for-pennies-a-gallon.aspx
29) http://curezone.com/blogs/fm.asp?i=973738
30) http://www.benefits-of-honey.com/vinegar-and-honey.html
31) http://thehealthyeatingsite.com/benefits-of-apple-cider-vinegar/

Trade Publications and Patents

1) http://www.google.com/patents?hl=en&lr=&vid=USPAT8206763&id=1isfAgAAEBAJ&oi=fnd&dq=apple+cider+vinegar&printsec=abstract#v=onepage&q=apple%20cider%20vinegar&f=false
2) http://www.freepatentsonline.com/y2013/0004591.html
3) http://www.bobbyshealthyshop.co.uk/Apple-Cider-Vinegar-In-The-Home.php

4) http://www.bobbyshealthyshop.co.uk/Apple-Cider-Vinegar-In-The-Garden.php
5) http://www.bobbyshealthyshop.co.uk/Apple-Cider-Vinegar-For-Pets.php
6) http://www.versatilevinegar.org/usesandtips.html#1b
7) http://www.wineworks.co.uk/content/cider-making-made-easy/
8) http://bragg.com/products/bragg-organic-apple-cider-vinegar.html
9) http://www.clarksnutrition.com/promog/cluster.asp?cpid=61&storeID=2691B1FE187D41ACB869A85CA5957A0A
10) http://www.melrosehealth.com.au/health_products/Diet_Weight_Digestion/Apple_Cider_Vinegar.aspx
11) http://www.stockhealth.com.au/apple-cider-vinegar-for-farm-animals

Printed in Great Britain
by Amazon.co.uk, Ltd.,
Marston Gate.